SLIM DOWN WITHOUT THE GYM

Simple straightforward diet plan to achieve weight loss
without the gym which results to happy,perfect body and
healthy lifestyle

JESSE A KING

Agreements

Lawful NOTICE

The Publisher has strived to be pretty much as precise and complete as conceivable in the making of this report, despite the way that he warrants or addresses absolutely never that the items inside are exact because of the quickly changing nature of the Internet.

While all endeavors have been made to confirm data given in this distribution, the Publisher takes care of blunders, exclusions, or opposite translation of the topic thus. Any apparent affronts of explicit people, people groups, or associations are unexpected.

In viable counsel books, similar to whatever else throughout everyday life, there are no assurances of pay made. Perusers are advised to answer on their own judgment about their singular conditions to as needs be acted.

This book isn't planned for use as a wellspring of lawful, business, bookkeeping or monetary guidance. All perusers are educated to look for administrations concerning able experts in lawful, business, bookkeeping and money fields.

You are urged to print this book for simple perusing.

Table of Contents

Foreword

There are lots of motivations behind why hefty or overweight individuals attempt to get more fit. A need to be better, to feel and look much improved while others need to have more energy to achieve their day to day undertakings.

Not a great explanation is, sound weight the board and fruitful weight reduction rely upon reasonable objectives as well as assumptions. Assuming you put forth objectives for yourself, it isn't difficult to meet them and get the opportunity to keep up with your weight.
Anybody can shed pounds actually. Get to know all your required data here.

Effective Weight Loss

Chapter 1:

Weight reduction Resolutions Basics

Weight reduction is the term that is on many individuals' psyches. A few need it for clinical reasons and others for tasteful purposes.

While there are numerous arrangements accessible in the present market and counsel can be found effectively over the web, accomplishing weight reduction objectives is absolutely an alternate matter. Individuals battle to shed pounds primarily in light of wrong assumption and misguidance because of the different item showcasing.

Before you rush and begin your weight reduction plan, think about the weight reduction rudiments first.

The Basics of Weight Loss

Diminishing one's pounds is one part of a compelling and fruitful weight reduction. The fact that everyone can connect with makes this the fundamental thought. It is additionally quantifiable and can bring noticeable outcomes. The words "weight reduction" convey these thoughts.

Getting in shape rotates on different significant viewpoints including reestablishing and working on one's well being, remaining on the track to accomplish all your weight reduction objectives, and changing and keeping a more streamlined body. For you to accomplish fruitful weight reduction, you need to remember the weight reduction essential standards. These incorporate the accompanying:

- Lose fat
- Remain roused
- Acquire muscle

For you to find actual success, you need to observe that you want to put forth additional attempts as there's no alternate way in shedding those undesirable pounds of yours.

Lose Fat: Diets Can Help You

Eating a right and solid adjusted diet is significant while getting more fit. Pick and follow an eating regimen that is wealthy in fiber and protein and low in refined carbs.

Whenever you have expanded your intake of fiber and protein, you will lose your weight slowly and your solid muscles will create. Likewise, assuming you consume less refined starches, you dispose of heaping calories, which don't give the required supplements of your body.

Acquire Muscles: Do Some Workouts

While shedding pounds, acquiring muscle can help. It is on the grounds that fat will be scorched to give you the right energy in which muscles expect in remaining alive. It's intriguing to note that a pound of fat requires just three calories while a pound of muscle needs 75-150 calories consistently to work. Thus, if you need to get results while shedding pounds, you must do exercises.

You can think about any activities or exercises. In any case, anaerobic and oxygen consuming activities are fundamental for your body to work harder. For improved results, change your work-out schedules to keep up with the excitement of your body.

Some consider get-healthy plans just to do exercises. There are even other people who select a rec center class. You don't have to burn through an immense measure of cash while doing exercises. You can do exercises at your home. Simply pick those activities that won't need exercise center hardware.

While doing exercises, treat it in a serious way and stick to your arrangement. Figure out how to be spurred. Practicing routinely with consistency and

responsibility is an unquestionable requirement. Try not to commit errors and expect for fast outcomes like the vast majority do. You need to observe that it additionally requires investment to get results.

Remaining Motivated

It is fundamental to acknowledge that weight reduction doesn't occur rapidly. Shedding pounds is an excursion wherein you really want to screen your advancement. With this, you will actually want to get results while being inspired with your arrangement.

Getting more fit might be simple for some in light of utilizing enhancement pills. Be that as it may, work on your general wellbeing and keep a solid weight, then stay propelled and get moving as this can have an effect.

Chapter 2:

Use Walks

Anybody can have the option to get in shape contingent upon the force and term of their strolling along with their eating regimen. That is the justification for why numerous specialists encouraged overweight individuals to involve strolls as this can be an extraordinary piece of their weight reduction venture. In any case, this doesn't imply that you really want to quit eating a solid adjusted diet. You actually need to adhere to your weight reduction plan. Strolling is only a reward for the people who need to get about no time.

Strolling As a Bonus to Your Weight Loss Journey

Certain individuals say that proactive tasks like strolling are not significant while attempting to get in shape. Yet, truly, involving strolls for your weight reduction can help you show up at your ideal outcomes.

Assuming you consider adding 30 minutes of energetic strolling to your everyday action, you would consume around 150 calories day to day. For you to lose a pound consistently, you want to dispose of 500 calories every day. Obviously, the more you invest your energy strolling and the speedier your speed is, you will actually want to consume more calories.

For you to find lasting success to get in shape through strolling, you want to keep up with the power of your activity at a vivacious or moderate level. With regards to weight reduction, the more you walk or the more extraordinary your strolling exercise is, the more calories you'll consume. In any case, you need to observe that equilibrium is fundamental.

In the event that you are new to active work and ordinary activity, you can begin at a low power and increment it progressively. Whenever you have prevailed with regards to getting in shape, you shouldn't eliminate your strolling practices in your day to day daily schedule as this will assist you with keeping up with your weight. Truly, studies showed that individuals who are keeping up with their weight for long haul generally think about standard strolls. Thus, continue to walk and guarantee to follow a sound adjusted diet.

Guide On How to Use Walking For Your Weight Loss

As referenced before, strolling alone won't assist you with shedding pounds effectively. You actually need to consider eating a sound eating routine as this can allow you to accomplish all your weight reduction objectives.

The vast majority who are attempting to get thinner find it hard to remain on the course. Through this aid, you will be spurred into getting in shape.

1. Follow along on Your Diet

The best key for you to try not to gorge is to stay focused on the thing you are eating. It might appear to be a basic undertaking, yet dealing with your eating regimen can be challenging. To demolish your weight reduction objectives, then, at that point, make a record of what you eat or drink. Tracking the calories of your food sources can likewise be really smart. Along these lines, you will actually want to keep up with your weight.

2. Measure Your Walks

There are various ways of observing your strolls or how far you have strolled. Following distance will permit you to look at courses and can help you in expanding your distance that can likewise allow you to consume more calories, which is significant assuming you're strolling to shed additional pounds of yours.

3. Keep a Walking Log

Keeping a mobile log is additionally significant like having a food log. This will assist you with being roused in getting in shape. Other than that, your strolling log will permit you to keep tabs on your development as you steadily increment the force of your strolls.

Chapter 3:

Use Fruits Rich in Vitamin C

Ongoing examinations propose that you will find success with your weight reduction assuming you will eat all the new citrus and a few vegetables and natural products that are plentiful in Vitamin C. It doesn't imply that Vitamin C is the new marvel drug for weight reduction, however specialists have found that consuming a deficient measure of Vitamin might frustrate one to get thinner.

Getting to Know More about Vitamin C

L-ascorbic acid isn't only useful in battling colds. In the event that you really want to get more fit for any reason, this nutrient can help you. Did you have any idea that natural products that are high in Vitamin C can allow you to consume more fats?

What Is Vitamin C?

L-ascorbic acid is additionally alluded to as an ascorbic corrosive. It's a water-dissolvable nutrient with a cell reinforcement capability in one's body. This simply implies that this kills free revolutionaries, which can harm cells.

Nutrients that are water-solvent are not put away in one's body. With this, you want to think about taking a new inventory of these consistently. If not, you will be in danger of fostering a lack that can prompt some medical problems after some time. Sadly, one's body doesn't have the ability of delivering Vitamin C. Thus, it is critical to guarantee that you take this supplement enough.

L-ascorbic acid and Weight Loss

Assuming you consider squeezing recipes for your weight reduction, you will obtain results assuming you will incorporate organic products that are plentiful in Vitamin C.

Scientists are looking for foods grown from the ground plentiful in Vitamin C that can expand your pace of consuming fats

Chapter 4:

Change Out Trans Fat For Healthier Fats

For a very long time, specialists and supplements have taught that low-fat eating regimens are the best key to effective weight reduction, forestalling medical conditions, and overseeing cholesterol.

To that end it is fundamental for you to have thoughts regarding changing out trans fat (terrible fat) to better fat. It is on the grounds that terrible fats can build your wellbeing and take a chance while great fats can safeguard your general medical issue. Better fats mean a lot to close to home and actual wellbeing, as a matter of fact.

Wipe out Trans Fats From Your Diet

Trans fats are typical fat particles that have been contorted as well as disfigured during a cycle, which is called hydrogenation. In this cycle, fluid vegetable oil is joined and warmed with hydrogen gas. To some degree, vegetable oils that are hydrogenated will make them less inclined to ruin and more steady, which is really great for all food producers and not something beneficial for you particularly on the off chance that you are keeping a sound weight.

Trans fats are not beneficial. Indeed, even a modest quantity of them is undesirable. The purpose for it is that these fats add to a few significant medical conditions like malignant growth and coronary illness.

Trans Fats Sources

While discussing trans fats, many individuals consider margarine. Indeed, the facts really confirm that there are a few margarines that are stacked with these fats. In any case, the fundamental wellspring of trans fats in the Western weight control plans comes from nibble food varieties and monetarily arranged prepared food varieties.

- Prepared Goods - wafers, treats, pizza batter, pie outsides,biscuits, and different breads including burger buns.

- Nibble Foods - corn, treats, tortilla chips, potato, microwave or on the other hand bundled popcorn.
- Seared Foods - French fries, chicken strips, hard taco shells, doughnuts, and seared chicken.
- Pre-Mixed Products - flapjack blend, chocolate beverage blend, furthermore, cake blend.
- Strong Fats - semi-strong vegetable shortening and stick margarine.

Be a Trans Fat Detective

While looking for your month to month or week by week food varieties, consistently think about perusing the marks and look at on the off chance that there is a presence of trans fats in the fixings. There are a few food varieties that accompany no trans fats name, their fixings may be a suspect.

With regards to buying margarine, pick the adaptations like a delicate tub and guarantee that the items accompany no grams of this terrible fat. Assuming you are accustomed to eating out, put away bread rolls, a few prepared food varieties and seared food sources. Stay away from these food varieties except if your picked café doesn't utilize trans fat while setting up their dinners. Moreover, request the counter individual or waiter from what kind of oil used to cook the food varieties. Assuming they will utilize trans fats, you can request that they set up your food sources with olive oil all things being equal.

In the event that you dispose of trans fats effectively, keeping away from cheap food is something that you want to do. Most states don't have marking guidelines for quick food varieties. Truth be told, this can be publicized as sans cholesterol in the event that the food sources are cooked in vegetable oil.

Instructions to Choose Healthy Fats

With the various wellsprings of dietary fats, the choices can confound. Yet, the main concern is to go with the great fats, which will offer you lots of weight reduction and medical advantages.

In the event that you're worried about the strength of your heart or your weight, rather than staying away from fat in your eating routine, attempt to supplant the terrible fats like trans fats with better fats. This simply implies that you should supplant a portion of your meat with vegetables and beans with the utilization of olive oil.

- Take out Trans Fats from Your Diet. On the off chance that you are going to a supermarket, consistently look at the names for you to know how much trans fats of what you will eat. Also, limit inexpensive food.
- Limit Your Intake of Bad Fats Like Saturated Fats. You can restrict soaked fats through scaling back full-fat dairy items and red meat. The best option for red meat is fish, beans, nuts, and fish if conceivable. Also, change to low fat variants of milk or full-fat dairy food sources.
- Think about Eating Omega-3 Daily. The best wellsprings of Omega-3 are pecans, fish, canola oil, soybean oil, ground flax seeds, and flaxseed oil.

Is The Amount Of Fat Too Much?

How much fat that is a lot for keeping a solid weight relies upon your weight, age, way of life, and your general medical issue. In this way, on the off chance that you don't have the foggiest idea how you will gauge your fat admission, converse with certain specialists or make your own customized fat breaking point. With this, you can not restrict yourself, but rather additionally you will lose terrible fats steadily without the need to think about alternate ways. Besides, this can lead you to taking better fats.

Trans fats are not only one of the terrible fats that you ought to keep away from while shedding pounds. Soaked fats are likewise a sort of fat, which are tracked down in different creature items. Diminishing this awful fat can likewise allow you to accomplish weight reduction objectives really.

Chapter 5:

Reconstruct Your Mind about Portion Sizes

In weight reduction, eating the right part size is fundamental. Be that as it may, many individuals who are attempting to get thinner find it hard to control food segment sizes. Indeed, it is truly intense from the start. Yet, whenever you have figured out how to control it, you will actually want to roll out certain improvements on how you eat and will allow you to consider food divides a device to get more fit effectively and eat in a better manner.

Estimating every piece that passes on your lips might be inconceivable. In any case, it is smart to begin estimating refreshments and food varieties until you have the inclination for considering right piece sizes for you to get in shape.

With the large numbers of food sources out there, you may be shocked that a solitary serving or two servings can have an effect. Thus, figure out how to reconstruct your psyche about segment sizes as this can assume an immense part in weight reduction.

Understanding Portion Sizes

Individuals frequently relate serving sizes to how much specific food sources that are put on their plates like at eateries. Tragically, that is not which part measures are. As a rule, partitions that are served are not exactly the genuine serving size. That is the motivation behind why a track down is intense to control segment sizes.

Many individuals don't frequently gauge their food varieties in any event, when at home. Normally, they think about what one serving of food is. Because of this, some don't comprehend the significance of genuine piece size.

For you to find out about segment sizes, attempt to quantify the serving size of your food varieties. Along these lines, you can not handle your calorie admission, but rather likewise you figure out how to watch segment sizes.

Overall principle of Thumb When Placing Portions On Your Plate

There are different ways on how you have some control over segments. A portion of these are the accompanying:

- The size of a baseball or a clench hand of a lady is equivalent to a serving of leafy foods.
- An adjusted modest bunch is about equivalent to a half cup of pasta or cooked rice.

- The size of cards' deck is around three ounces of meat, which is a typical serving size.
- The huge egg's size or golf ball is around one-fourth cup of nuts. A PC mouse has a similar size to a little potato.

Beside those referenced ways, estimating is as yet viewed as the most ideal way to ensure that you are eating the right piece size. Whenever you've estimated your food varieties for the interim, you can ensure that you are getting the right serving size.

On the off chance that you don't know whether you got the right size, take a stab at putting less on your plate. Then, at that point, assuming that you are ravenous, go for a second half part for you certainly.

Chapter 6:

Alter Your Perspective on Salt and Use Fresh Herbs

Summary

Salt doesn't make your body lose or acquire fat. Indeed, salt has no measure of calories. Nonetheless, consuming high amounts of salt might result in transitory weight gain. It is on the grounds that this makes your body keep water. Then again, in the event that you polish off less salt, your body might lose some weight in light of the fact that your body ousts water.

It is somewhat fascinating to note that most accidents eat less carbs that brag speedy weight reduction rely upon food sources with no or minimal salt substance. In any case, this doesn't imply that you will eliminate salt on your eating routine. You can constantly salt in the event that you need to. Nonetheless, to see quick outcomes, why not utilize new spices rather than salt? Along these lines, you can get in shape, yet in addition you will have a better weight.

Why Change Your Mind about Salt?

Albeit salt is a fundamental piece of one's eating regimen, eating a lot of this can be unsafe. As a matter of fact, measurements show that a greater part of Americans eat an excess of salt. For your body to work appropriately, you want to shop for 500 mg every day.

What Sodium Does

Eliminating salt from your diet isn't required. Specialists actually encouraged weight watchers to involve this for your body to appropriately work. Sodium is a component that adjusts your body liquid, has an impact in compression as well as unwinding of muscles, and sends nerve motivations.

Be that as it may, a lot of measures of sodium in your eating regimen might have an adverse consequence in one's body. This holds and draws in water, which leads to an increased blood volume that makes your heart work harder than it used to be.

Involving Herbs For Your Weight Loss

In the present world, most food varieties found in the market are unfortunate. That is the justification for why you should be astute while looking for food sources that will suit your eating regimen and will lead you to weight reduction results. In the event that you assume you got the right fixings, including new spices your dish can have an effect.

There are lots of new species out there that you can utilize. Some of them include:

- Parsley
- Basil
- Oregano
- Cumin
- Thyme
- Rosemary
- Chives
- Dark pepper
- Nutmeg
- Cinnamon
- Paprika
- Stew Powder

Each of these can either be flavorful or zesty. There are a few that are sweet. There are spices, which can be matched with organic products for flavors and sound treats that will flavor your solid eating routine. These spices can be found without any problem. You can track them down at the closest nearby store in your space.

Getting everything rolling When Using Fresh Herbs

Certain individuals who are utilized to counterfeit food varieties could feel that adding these food sources can be challenging. Obviously, it very well may be hard to begin

with spices particularly on the off chance that you haven't thought about these sorts of food sources for quite a while. For you to find lasting success with these spices, here are a few hints that you might consider:

- Get Fresh Herbs. The fresher the spices, the more prominent the advantages will be. Dried spices actually have flavors, yet they don't accompany other solid ascribes. If you have any desire to utilize new spices, simply hack them into little pieces and afterward adhere to the guidelines on your own cookbook.

- Become Your Own. New spices are not as exorbitant as what other individuals think. To appreciate reserve funds and stay away from problems while shopping in a supermarket, then begin developing spices on your lawn. Through this, you can get a good deal on purchasing spices, yet additionally it will be a lot simpler for you to routinely cook your recipes.

Including new spices your eating routine is smart. Be that as it may, before you choose to add this, make a point to counsel your doctor first. The explanation for it is that there are certain individuals who have sensitivities with spices. Subsequently, if you would rather not face any burden while getting in shape, then, at that point, figure out which spices are the most ideal for you.

Chapter 7:

Change Your View about Whole Grains

An eating regimen that is wealthy in entire grains can assist in battling your paunch with swelling while at the same time diminishing the gamble of coronary illness.

Another review showed that individuals who followed health improvement plans, which consolidate entire grain breads and oats are probably going to accomplish weight reduction objectives effectively.

Moreover, those individuals who consider an entire grain diet encountered a drop of around 38% in CRP or C-receptor protein, which is an irritation's pointer in one's body that is connected to coronary illness.

Scientists said that the outcomes propose that considering entire grains into your weight reduction excursion can assist you with consuming fat and lessen the gamble of fostering a coronary illness.

Entire Grains Versus Refined Grains

In a new report, a gathering of corpulent individuals with metabolic disorder was separated into 2 gatherings. Metabolic condition is an assortment of the gamble factors, which increase the gamble of diabetes and coronary illness.

The two gatherings were encouraged to cut calories for a sum of 12 weeks. Be that as it may, one gathering was told to take just entire grains or entire grain items while the other was asked not to think about eating any entire grain food sources.

Toward the end, the two gatherings showed weight reduction achievement. Both have encountered a decline in their muscle to fat ratio. Be that as it may, individuals who have a place with the gathering who will eat entire grains just have decreased weight quickly. They additionally experienced different advantages. Yet, the people who have a place with the refined grain bunch didn't get different advantages.

Entire Grain Sources

In the event that you are looking for a wellspring of entire grain, here are the few entire grains you can consider:

- Entire wheat
- Cereal
- Popcorn
- Earthy colored rice
- Entire grain corn
- Millet
- Bulgur
- Triticale
- Wild rice
- Buckwheat
- Entire grain
- Sorghum
- Quinoa

There are likewise entire grains that you can add on your bites or dinners. These are:

- Entire grain cereals like toasted oat cereal
- Entire grain nibble chip
- Utilizing entire grain flour
- Popcorn

Entire Grains on the Food Labels

Assuming you are attempting to search for food varieties that contain entire grains, pick food sources that have the accompanying:

- Bulgur
- Oats
- Earthy colored rice
- Entire oats
- Wild rice
- Entire wheat
- Entire grain corn

On the off chance that you experience a few names, for example, "multi-grain", "wheat", "broken wheat", "seven-grain", "100 percent wheat", and soon, they don't ordinarily contain entire grains.

You need to observe that tone is the premise of entire grains. There are a few breads that can be brown in light of their fixings or molasses. Undoubtedly, actually look at the nourishment realities.

Chapter 8:

Remember the Water

Summary

There are different motivations behind why it is fundamental to hydrate while getting in shape. Hence, remember to hydrate as this can assist you with accomplishing all your weight reduction objectives.

Motivations behind Why You Should Not Forget Water for Your Weight Loss Resolution
One of the fundamental motivations behind why you should hydrate while slimming down is that this can assist you with keeping away from parchedness. Starting weight reduction is brought about by loss of water. You really want to stay hydrated.

The method involved with consuming fats and calories likewise requires an adequate stockpile of water for you to work productively. You need to remember that parchedness lessens the course of fat-consuming. When you have consumed calories, you make poisons like fumes emerging from your vehicle. Because of this, water assumes a significant part in flushing poisons out of your body.

On the off chance that you attempt weight reduction to assemble abs and muscles, water assists in keeping up with muscle tone through helping muscles in their capacity to agreement and this greases up your joints. With appropriate hydration, you will actually want to decrease muscle as well as joint irritation while working out.

Many individuals know that a sound weight reduction rotates around having a lot of fiber. Be that as it may, without water, your weight reduction won't ever find success as you would encounter stoppage.

Chapter 9:

Use Affirmations to Stay on Course

Affirmations can assist you with getting rolling. To that end it means quite a bit to involve certifications for you to keep on track. Through these, accomplishing all your weight reduction objectives is conceivable. All you want is to know what attestations are and how they can help you to be successful in getting thinner.

Affirmations Defined

Affirmations are essentially whatever you think or say. Individuals avow what they anticipate in life all the time with their convictions and contemplations. For example, assuming you accept that horrible weight is incomprehensible and troublesome, it will be. However, when you accept that it tends to be extreme yet you can accomplish it, then, at that point, it will certainly be. You need to remember that activities understand considerations. Along these lines, with positive assertions, your activities will likewise be positive, which will permit you to continue to push ahead.

Remaining on the course is never a simple occupation particularly assuming you are encircled with enticements. For that reason confirmations are helpful. Here are some of them:

- I will keep a solid adjusted diet.
- I will follow a specific diet. regimen that will work on my capacity to lose additional pounds.
- I will practice 1 hour consistently and 3 days every week.
- I will walk more to consume more calories.
- I will trail closely behind 6 dietary pattern.

Chapter 10:

The Benefits of Maintaining A Healthy Weight

The advantages of keeping a sound weight are quite a large number. It works on personal satisfaction, yet additionally it supports one's life.

Here are the principal advantages of keeping a sound weight:

Uneasiness Relief

At the point when somebody needs to convey additional pounds, their dynamic way of life is likewise impacted. In any event, losing 5-10% of your weight will support lessening different throbs as well as torments that are related to not being dynamic.

The additional pounds of your body might cause more burdens on the bones, muscles, and joints, which will make them capability harder than ordinary just to move around. Yet, on the off chance that your weight is less, your body will actually want to work productively and will stay away from harm, which can block an individual from effectively doing their everyday exercises.

Better Heart

Assuming your weight is high, your heart probably won't have the option to take care of its responsibilities successfully regardless of whether you are resting. Notwithstanding, on the off chance that you keep a solid weight, how much blood that is going to different crucial organs of the body will expand, which will likewise permit your heart to productively take care of its business.

Keeping a solid weight likewise diminishes stresses on the heart and decreases one's gamble of coronary failure, angina, and hypertension.

Lower Risk of Diabetes

Based on a few examinations and studies, overweight individuals are at a more serious gamble to experience the ill effects of Diabetes Type II. In the event that you have previously determined to have this ailment, it is vital to shed pounds as this will permit you to control it in a superior manner. In the event that you don't have this condition, keeping a solid weight will diminish the dangers of Diabetes.

Cancer growth Avoidance

Specialists said that weight reduction assumes an enormous part to dispose of disease. Getting in shape won't simply forestall disease improvement, yet additionally this can decrease the chance of creating different sorts of cancer growth that are known these days. As per a few examinations, overweight ladies are more probable inclined to gallbladder, bosom, uterine, colon, cervical, and ovary disease while overweight men might foster prostate, rectal, and colon cancer growth.

Osteoarthritis is a condition where patients experience the ill effects of joint paints. Because of overabundant weight, many individuals may be in danger of fostering this condition. Notwithstanding, with a kept up with sound weight, this issue can be forestalled effectively before it will begin. Alongside practice and a sound eating regimen, the body joints will convey decreased weight and will forestall harm after some time.

These are just a portion of the various advantages of keeping a solid body weight. In this way, to live better and keep away from some illnesses, begin getting thinner at this point.